A PROGRAMMED SURGERY MANUAL

Fluids and Electrolytes

MW00984660

PETER R. KASTL, WILLIAM P. COLEMAN, III, M.D., THEODORE DRAPANAS, M.D., AND ROBERT F. RYAN, M.D.

Department of Surgery, Section of Plastic Surgery, Tulane University
School of Medicine, New Orleans, Louisiana

series editor: Robert F. Ryan, M.D.

APPLETON-CENTURY-CROFTS / New York
A Publishing Division of Prentice-Hall, Inc.

75 76 77 78 79 / 10 9 8 7 6 5 4 3 2 1

Library of Congress Catalog Card Number:
75-18388

Printed in the United States of America
0-8385-7882-9

ACKNOWLEDGMENTS

The authors are indebted to Virginia Zachert, Ph.D., and Preston Lea Wildes, M.D., of the Learning Materials Division, Department of Obstetrics and Gynecology, Medical College of Georgia, and Stuart R. Johnson, Ph.D., and Rita B. Johnson, Ph.D., of the Self-Instructional Materials Project, Southern Medical School Consortium, for their advice and help in preparing this material. We also wish to thank Robert F. Mager, Ph.D., for his constant inspiration and encouragement.

The authors are indebted to Ms. Betsy Ewing, medical illustrator, for the drawings used in this text. For typing and proofreading of the manuscript, the authors wish to thank Mrs. Gertrude Burguieres.

CONTENTS

INTRODUCTION

This short text is designed to teach medical students during their clinical blocks to recognize fluid-electrolyte disorders and to formulate a daily fluid and electrolyte plan for maintenance as well as correction purposes.

Students must have adequate preparation in the basic sciences before beginning. Please note that this text is not all-encompassing and that controversial material is often simplified.

From studies on self-teaching from programmed texts, it has been shown that filling in the blanks provides better comprehension and retention of the material than thinking or reciting the answers. The authors therefore recommend that the student fill in each blank with pen or pencil before checking the answer on the following page.

A posttest is supplied at the end of the text. The student is advised to test comprehension immediately after completing the material.

SOURCE MATERIAL

Because the continuity of a programmed instruction text tends to be disrupted by footnotes and references, each item has not been individually annotated. Instead, the references on which the factual material is based are listed below:

Beeson PB, McDermott W (eds): Cecil-Loeb Textbook of Medicine, 13th ed. Philadelphia, Saunders, 1971

Diem K, Lentner C (eds): Scientific Tables, 7th ed. Basel, Switzerland, CIBA-Geigy, 1970

McGilvery RW: Biochemistry, a Functional Approach. Philadelphia, Saunders, 1970

Sabiston DC Jr (ed): Davis-Christopher Textbook of Surgery, 10th ed. Philadelphia, Saunders, 1972

Scribner BH (ed): Fluid and Electrolyte Balance. Seattle, University of Washington, 1953

PART I

Basic Considerations

(Frame 1)

A glance at a globe reveals that the world is mostly water. Man, too, is composed mainly of _Water_ .

The average adult male is 60 percent water, which is concentrated mostly in muscle tissue.

10. (continued)

A. Start infusion at 8 AM. Even if behind schedule, infuse no faster than 1 liter every 2 hours (or 150 drops per minute).

B. No. 1—1 liter D5W; add 20 mEq KCl and 50 mEq NH_4 Cl; in by 10 AM to 12 noon
No. 2—1 liter D5NS; in by 2 to 4 PM
No. 3—same as No. 1; in by 6 to 8 PM
No. 4—same as No. 2; in by 10 PM to 12 midnight
No. 5—1 liter D5W; add 20 mEq KCl; in by 2 to 4 AM
No. 6—1 liter D5W; in by 6 to 8 AM

(Frame 136)

water

Since 1 liter of water is equivalent to 1 kg, a 75 kg average male contains (75 × 0.6 =) _____45. 0_____ liters of water. Remember that this water is concentrated mostly in ___muscle_____ tissue.

10.

Bottle	Water	Na⁺	Cl⁻	K⁺
1. (D5W)	1,000		70 (NH_4Cl)	20 (KCl)
2. (D5NS)	1,000	150	150	
3. (D5W)	1,000		70	20
4. (D5NS)	1,000	150	150	
5. (D5W)	1,000		20	20
6. (D5W)	1,000			
	6,000	300	460	60

(Frame 135)

The table in the following frame is included for reference only. Skim over it and notice the differences in percentage of body water between infants and adults, and between the forms of body habitus.

9. combines saline depletion and water excess
saline

10. After totaling a patient's fluid and electrolyte needs for the next 24 hours, you find that he needs 6 liters water, 300 mEq Na^+, 500 mEq Cl^-, and 65 mEq K^+. Included in this is 100 mEq NH_4Cl (should be given in two 50 mEq doses). Devise a plan for the administration of these fluids and electrolytes, and order it, beginning at 8 AM.

(Frame 134)

BODY WATER AS PERCENTAGE OF BODY WEIGHT

Habitus	Infant	Adult Male	Adult Female
Thin	80%	65%	55%
Average	70	60	50
Obese	65	55	45

(Frame 5)

8. NH_4

9. A high school football player is brought to your office, unconscious. He collapsed 20 minutes after practice was over, having drunk an unknown quantity of water. The diagnosis is _____

_____ and the treatment is

_____ administration.

(Frame 133)

Simple calculation thus yields the amount of total body ___WATER___.
The patient's weight in pounds is converted to kilograms by dividing the weight by 2.2. An obese female of 242 lb weighs $242/2.2 =$ ___110___ kg. Referring to the previous table, then, one can see that her body contains $110 \times 0.45 =$ _____ liters of water.

$$\begin{array}{r} 1\,1\,0, \\ 2.2\overline{)2\,4\,2.0,} \\ 2\,2 \\ \hline 2\,2 \end{array}$$

$$\begin{array}{r} 110 \\ \times .45 \\ \hline \end{array}$$

7. high

   metabolic alkalosis
   (K^+ and Cl^- depletion)

8. For a challenge: if the preceding patient had normal values for Cl^- and K^+, yet was still alkalotic, you would treat him with 100 mEq of _____ Cl.

(Frame 132)

water
110
49.5

How much water does the body of a 242 lb obese male contain? (Refer to table on Frame 5.) _____

5. 40
6. dextrose

7. Laboratory data on patient E.B. are: Na^+ = 139; Cl^- = 91; HCO_3^- = 34; K^+ = 3.1. Based on the high HCO_3^- and the low K^+ and Cl^-, you would expect the pH to be ______________ (high/low). Give a diagnosis.
____

(Frame 131)

$$(242/2.2) \times 0.55 = 60.5 \text{ liters}$$

The total body water can be subdivided by a "rule of thirds" into several fluid compartments. First, one-third is extracellular; two-thirds is intracellular (but less so in people with less _____ tissue).

(Frame 8)

3. Saline
4. pH

5. IV fluids should never contain more than _____ mEq/liter K⁺.
6. All IV fluids should be ordered 5 percent with _____ .

muscle

Second, of the extracellular water, one-third is intravascular (plasma water) and two-thirds is interstitial. The "rule of thirds" is summarized by the block diagrams in Frames 10 and 11.

1. osmolality
2. Na$^+$

3. (Water/Saline) affects primarily the extracellular fluid compartment.
4. Of the common laboratory determinations, serum _____ best displays changes in acid-base status.

(Frame 129)

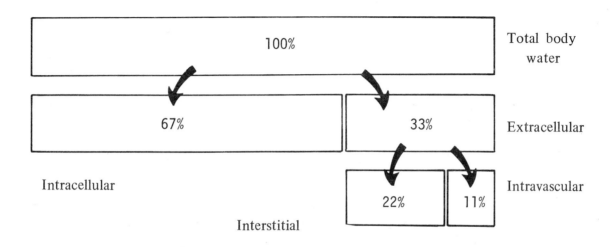

	Total body water
100%	

67%	33%
Intracellular	Extracellular

	22%	11%
Interstitial		Intravascular

(Frame 10)

1. Water moves rapidly among the various fluid compartments so as to standardize
   _____ .

2. Of the common laboratory determinations, serum _____
   best displays changes in osmolality.

(Frame 128)

Fill in the blanks:

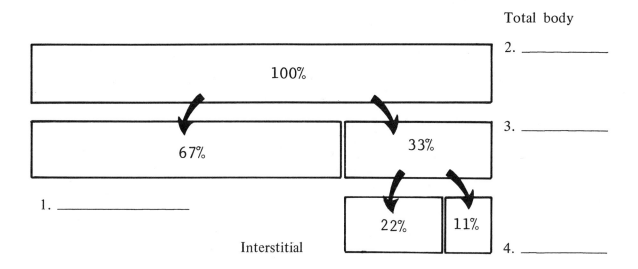

Total body

2. _____

100%

3. _____

67%   33%

1. _____

22%   11%

Interstitial   4. _____

(Frame 11)

POSTTEST

What have you learned?

(Frame 127)

1. Intracellular
2. water
3. Extracellular
4. Intravascular

The plasma volume of a normal 75 kg man is calculated as follows:

1. 75 kg × 0.6 = 45 liters total body water
2. 45 liters total body water = 30 liters intracellular
                               15 liters extracellular
3. 15 liters extracellular water = 10 liters interstitial
                                    5 liters intravascular

(Frame 12)

One last tip is that in a 24-hour continuous infusion, 10 mg heparin and 1 mg hydrocortisone in each bottle of fluid will extend the life of the vein being used by preventing clotting and reducing phlebitis.

(Frame 126)

The most important concept of this book is that water rapidly distributes throughout all fluid compartments. In other words, a 3 liter addition to total body water results in the addition of 2 liters to the intracellular compartment and 1 liter to the _____ compartment.

(Frame 13)

dextrose

Do not add too many different electrolytes to the same bottle, so as to avoid any chemical interactions (eg, formation of $CaCO_3$, a precipitate). Always remember the rules on giving K^+.

extracellular ("rule of thirds")

The normal 75 kg man of two frames ago would then have 32 liters of intracellular and 16 liters of extracellular water. Of course, of the 1 liter added to the extracellular compartment, two-thirds becomes interstitial and one-third becomes _____.

The hardest part of this patient evaluation program is the fluid plan formulation. First decide how much saline you can give and then make all fluids 5 percent with

_____ .

(Frame 124)

intravascular

Water behaves in such a manner because there are particles of solute dissolved in every fluid compartment; the osmolality or concentration of these particles is standardized throughout the body by this rapid movement of water.

(Frame 15)

No. 6—same as No. 4; in by 9 to 11 PM
No. 7—1 liter D5 1/2NS; add 20 mEq KCl; in by 1 to 3 AM
No. 8—same as No. 2; in by 4 to 6 AM
No. 9—same as No. 4; in by 6 to 8 AM

The time was less rigidly ordered in the early morning so as to minimize activity in the ward. Even if the fluids were given behind schedule, the next morning's reevaluation would make up for any lack.

Therefore, measurement of osmolality in one compartment indicates the
_____ of all other compartments. In clinical medicine, osmolality is
most easily measured in the blood (the _____ compartment).

(Frame 16)

Here is how the order would read:

1. Start infusion at 8 AM. Even if behind schedule, infuse no faster than 1 liter every 2 hours (or 150 drops per minute)
2. No. 1—1 liter D5NS; add 20 mEq KCl; in by 10 to 11 AM
   No. 2—1 liter D5W; in by 12 to 1 PM
   No. 3—same as No. 1; in by 2 to 3 PM
   No. 4—1 liter D5W; add 20 mEq KCl, in by 4 to 5 PM
   No. 5—same as No. 1; in by 6 to 7 PM

(Frame 122)

osmolality
intravascular

The particles in the extracellular space which determine its osmolality are almost exclusively ions, consisting of three major types:

1. Sodium (Na^+)—130 to 145 mEq/liter in serum
2. Chloride (Cl^-)—100 to 110 mEq/liter in serum
3. Bicarbonate (HCO_3^-)—25 to 30 mEq/liter in serum

(Frame 17)

dextrose

The fluid order should be written showing the approximate time of each liter's infusion and indicating explicitly what is to be in each bottle (remember the rules regarding K^+).

(Frame 121)

Because sodium is the major ion in the extracellular space, it is largely responsible for the extracellular volume as well as its osmolality. Sodium exerts most of the extracellular osmotic pull attracting water.

Note that the totals did not come out exactly as the calculated allowances, but a good approximation is all that is desired. Note also that all fluid is 5 percent with

_____ .

Other ions can also affect osmolality, eg, ketones in diabetic ketoacidosis or SO_4^{2-} and PO_4^{3-} in uremia.

However, these abnormal states will not be covered in this book.

Bottle No.	Water	Na$^+$	Cl	K$^+$
1 (D5NS)	1,000	150	170	20 (KCl)
2 (D5W)	1,000			
3 (D5NS)	1,000	150	170	20
4 (D5W)	1,000		20	20
5 (D5NS)	1,000	150	170	20
6 (D5W)	1,000		20	20
7 (D5 1/2NS)	1,000	75	95	20
8 (D5W)	1,000			
9 (D5W)	1,000		20	20
	9,000	525	665	140

(Frame 119)

Rule No. 1: Serum sodium (Na^+) concentration measures essentially one-half serum osmolality (as well as the _____ of the other fluid compartments).

KCl comes in small vials of 20 and 40 mEq in 20 ml water (negligible volume), so plan to add appropriate amounts to every other liter of fluid. One way to give the desired electrolytes is shown in the following frame.

osmolality

Rule No. 2: Always check laboratory results for error, as follows: $Cl^- + HCO_3^- + 10 = Na^+$ (the number 10 is derived from the contribution of minor anions). In fact, this check is the primary reason for obtaining a serum chloride determination.

(Frame 21)

Four liters of normal saline might overload his circulatory system. The other fluid used is 5 percent dextrose in water.

Abbreviations: 5 percent dextrose in water—D5W

5 percent dextrose in normal saline—D5NS

5 percent dextrose in one-half normal saline—D5 1/2NS

(Frame 117)

Here are some laboratory results: Na^+, 140; Cl^-, 105; HCO_3, 25. By rule No. 1, osmolality equals approximately _____ . By rule No. 2, $Cl^- + HCO_3 + 10 = Na^+$, so there is no laboratory error.

To translate amounts of electrolyte into an order, first determine how much saline you can give (1 liter saline contains 150 mEq NaCl). Keep in mind that some Cl^- is to be given as KCl.

For this patient, you can give 3 liters saline (= 450 mEq NaCl) and 1 liter one-half normal saline (= 75 mEq NaCl), so that he receives 4 liters water and 525 mEq NaCl.

(Frame 116)

Rule No. 3:   Never confuse "sodium" with "saline." "Sodium" is a laboratory measurement done to determine the _____ of the bodily fluid compartments. "Saline" is a fluid used as therapy under certain conditions.

(Frame 23)

In formulating the actual fluid plan, one must resolve always to order all fluids with 5 percent dextrose, because 1 liter of this solution gives a patient 200 calories he would not otherwise receive.

(Frame 115)

osmolality

One further concept:

Remember that the rapid movement of water standardizes _____
in all fluid compartments.

(Frame 24)

MAINTENANCE ALLOWANCES

	Volume (ml/day)	Na^+ (mEq)	Cl^- (mEq)	K^+ (mEq)
Urine	1,500	50	90	40
Insensible	1,000	0	0	0
Gastric	3,000	135	270	30
TOTAL	5,500	185	360	70

CORRECTION ALLOWANCES

	Volume (ml/day)	Na^+ (mEq)	Cl^- (mEq)	K^+ (mEq)
Water	1,000			
Saline	2,000	300	300	
Acid-base				
Potassium			74	74
OVERALL TOTAL	8,500	485	734	144

(Frame 114)

osmolality

A 3 liter addition of water to the extracellular space was said to have enlarged the 30 liter and 15 liter intra- and extracellular compartments of a 75 kg average male to 32 liters and 16 liters, respectively. A 3 liter addition of isosmotic saline enlarges only the extracellular compartment to 18 liters and does not enter the intracellular compartment.

(Frame 25)

4. Potassium—serum K^+ is low. K^+ capacity is 45 mEq/kg $\times$ 66 kg = 2,970 mEq. From nomogram in Frame 83, there is about a 5 percent depletion; therefore, add 0.05 $\times$ 2,970 $\times$ 1/2 = 74 mEq to K^+ and Cl^- columns.

The total amounts of electrolytes to be added are shown in the next frame.

(Frame 113)

This result is not surprising if one considers that normal saline possesses the same osmolality as blood and is already "standardized" to the _____ of the other fluid compartments. Thus no movement of water between the fluid compartments occurs.

3. Acid-base—pH is 7.50 (high). From nomogram, P_{CO_2} is 44 (normal). HCO_3^- is 33 (metabolic alkalosis); however, check for a low K^+ (it is low: 3.2)—skip to potassium to see if there is depletion.

(Frame 112)

osmolality

Therefore, by administering intravenous saline to a patient, one immediately increases his blood volume by one-third the delivered amount (the other two-thirds becomes interstitial). The main intracellular ions are potassium (K^+) and phosphate, which are mainly responsible for intracellular osmolality.

(Frame 27)

For correction allowances, proceed in proper order:

1. Water—Na^+ is high, so add 1,000 ml water to that column.
2. Saline—Δ ECV $= -5 + (0.3 \times 5) + (148 - 140)/148 \times (0.4 \times 71)$
   $$= -5 + 1.5 + 1.5$$
   $$= -2 \text{ liters (saline depletion)}$$

Therefore, add 2,000 ml to water column and 300 mEq to Na^+ and Cl^-.

(Frame 111)

SUMMARY

1. Total body water is distributed in several fluid compartments.
2. Water moves rapidly and freely among these compartments to standardize the _____ or concentration of dissolved particles.
3. Sodium, chloride, and bicarbonate determine extracellular osmolality.
4. Potassium and phosphate determine _____ osmolality.

Maintenance allowances are thus:

	Water	Na^+	Cl^-	K^+
Urine	1,500 ml	50 mEq	90 mEq	40 mEq
Insensible	1,000	0	0	0
Gastric	3,000	135	270	30
TOTAL	5,500	185	360	70

(Frame 110)

osmolality
intracellular

(Frame 29)

To begin figuring his fluid and electrolyte needs, first check for laboratory error:

$$105 \ (Cl^-) + 33 \ (HCO_3^-) + 10 = 148 \ (Na^+).$$

For maintenance allowances, enter values for urine and insensible losses as shown in Frame 99. For gastric allowance, volume = 3,000 ml water; $Cl^- = 90$ mEq/liter $\times$ 3 liters = 270 mEq; $Na^+ = 1/2 \times 270$ (pH < 4) = 135 mEq; $K^+ = 10$ mEq/liter $\times$ 3 liters = 30 mEq.

(Frame 109)

PART II

Saline and Water Imbalances

(Frame 30)

A 50-year-old man was transferred to your ward after having undergone surgery five days ago for a perforated gastric ulcer. At the time of operation, he weighed 71 kg but now weighs 66 kg. In the last 24 hours, his gastric suction has removed 3 liters of fluid, pH = 3.5 and $Cl^- = 90$ mEq/liter. His electrolyte picture now is $Na^+ = 148$; $Cl^- = 105$; $HCO_3^- = 33$; $K^+ = 3.2$; pH = 7.50. At operation, $Na^+ = 140$.

(Frame 108)

Saline and water behave differently in the body. As discussed before, water equilibrates into all fluid compartments, whereas _____ stays in the extracellular compartment.

Note from the preceding plan that water depletion is treated with 1 liter of water; saline depletion, with the appropriate amount of saline (1 liter saline contains 150 mEq NaCl); metabolic alkalosis, with 100 mEq NH_4Cl; and potassium depletion, with KCl. This plan is complicated and is best illustrated with an example.

saline

That is, water imbalances are total body water imbalances; saline imbalances are confined to the extracellular compartment. Which kind of imbalance (water or saline) do you think would affect osmolality? _____ _____

2. Determine percentage of K^+ depletion or excess (Frame 82). If excess, obtain EKG; if this is abnormal, give IV calcium gluconate and call for help.

3. If there is K^+ depletion, calculate correction (Frame 84) and record one-half this number in both K^+ and Cl^- columns, indicating KCl to be given.

IV. Construct fluid plan after totaling entries.

(Frame 106)

water imbalance (saline is isosmotic)

The diagram in the following frame depicts a 3 liter saline excess and a 3 liter saline depletion in a normal 75 kg man. Note that Na^+ concentration and, therefore, osmolality are unchanged in either case.

2. If pH low, check HCO_3^- (25 to 30): if low (metabolic acidosis), calculate correction (Frame 67) and add this number to Na^+ column, indicating that this amount of $NaHCO_3$ will be given. If HCO_3^- normal but P_{CO_2} high (respiratory acidosis), obtain adequate ventilation.
3. If pH high, check HCO_3^-: if high (metabolic alkalosis) check first for K^+ depletion; if none, add 100 mEq to Cl^- column, indicating that 100 mEq of NH_4Cl will be given.

E. Potassium correction
1. If K^+ (3.8 to 4.4) is abnormal, determine K^+ capacity (Frame 81).

SALINE IMBALANCES

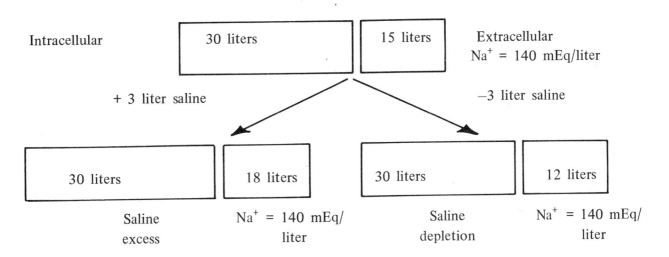

Intracellular

30 liters   15 liters

Extracellular
Na^+ = 140 mEq/liter

+ 3 liter saline

−3 liter saline

30 liters   18 liters   30 liters   12 liters

Saline
excess

Na^+ = 140 mEq/
liter

Saline
depletion

Na^+ = 140 mEq/
liter

(Frame 34)

C. Saline correction—check for signs of saline imbalance
   1. Calculate change in ECV (Frame 49); if positive, enter nothing (consider diuretics); if negative, enter 1,000 ml water and 150 mEq in Na^+ and Cl^- columns for each liter of saline depletion.
D. Acid-base correction
   1. pH should be 7.35 to 7.45; if altered, obtain P_{CO_2} (35 to 45) from nomogram (Frame 59).

(Frame 104)

The diagram in the next frame shows a 3 liter water excess and a 3 liter water depletion in the same 75 kg man. Note that Na^+ concentration (osmolality) has changed.

(Frame 35)

III. Calculate Correction allowances
   A. Get body weight; hematocrit; serum Na^+, K^+, Cl^-, HCO_3^-, pH; check lab report for error (Frame 21).
   B. Water correction—check for signs of water imbalance
      1. Na^+ should be 130 to 145: if high, enter 1,000 ml in water column; if low, enter nothing.

(Frame 103)

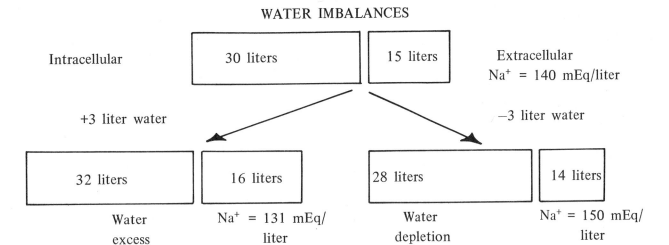

WATER IMBALANCES

(Frame 36)

Here is the program for fluid therapy:

    I. Day begins
   II. Calculate maintenance allowances
       A. If gastric suction, get 24 hour report (volume, pH, Cl^- concentration).
       B. Calculate maintenance allowances (Frame 100) and record them on the fluid form (Frame 98).

(Frame 102)

Water imbalances are easier to diagnose, because they always involve a change in serum Na^+ concentration (osmolality).

Water depletion is defined as an increase in serum Na^+, whereas water excess is defined as a _____ .

Do not get the Na^+ in the previous frame confused with its serum concentration (Frame 23); Na^+ and Cl^- are administered as saline (1 liter of normal saline contains 150 mEq NaCl).

For gastric losses, Cl^- and K^+ are calculated by multiplying 100 (or measured Cl^- concentration) and 10 times the previous day's volume in liters. Na^+ is figured from Cl^- and is pH dependent.

(Frame 101)

decrease in serum Na^+

Hematocrit does not change in water imbalances, because the red cells are part of the total fluid compartment and swell or shrink in the same proportion as the plasma compartment.

Hemoglobin, though, is an absolute quantity and changes in the same manner as the Na^+ concentration: high in water _____ , low in water _____ . Hemoglobin normally is 14 to 18 g.

(Frame 38)

Maintenance allowances are as follows:

	Water	Na^+	Cl^-	K^+
Urine	1,500 ml/day	50 mEq	90 mEq	40 mEq
Insensible (skin, lung)	1,000	0	0	0
Gastric	previous volume	pH>4: same as Cl^- pH<4: 1/2 Cl^-	100 mEq/liter or measured	10 mEq/liter

depletion
excess

Keep in mind that the intracellular compartment takes two-thirds of the brunt of the imbalance. Thus, either a severe water depletion or a severe excess will cause cerebral dysfunction by shrinking or swelling the brain cells.

(Frame 39)

The fluids actually given include saline, dextrose in water, NH_4Cl, KCl, and $NaHCO_3$. Preparation of a fluid plan will be discussed later.

Other symptomatology of water imbalances are:

1. Depletion—thirst, concentrated urine
2. Excess—oliguira (due to major surgery, cardiac failure, blood loss)

Treatment of a water imbalance is simply to give or restrict water for depletion or excess, respectively.

MAINTENANCE ALLOWANCES

	Volume (ml/day)	Na$^+$(mEq)	Cl$^-$(mEq)	K$^+$(mEq)
Urine				
Insensible (skin, lung)				
Gastric				
TOTAL				

CORRECTION ALLOWANCES

	Volume (ml/day)	Na$^+$(mEq)	Cl$^-$(mEq)	K$^+$(mEq)
Water				
Saline				
Acid-base				
Potassium				
OVERALL TOTAL				

(Frame 98)

Saline imbalances are less easily diagnosed, since they involve only the _____ fluid compartment and the osmolality is unchanged.

24
maintenance
saline
potassium

    After maintenance and correction allowances are totaled, they are then translated into a viable fluid plan. The actual form on which to record these allowances is given in the next frame.

(Frame 97)

extracellular

In saline depletion, there usually is a history of loss of sodium-containing fluid (vomiting, diarrhea, sweating), and there are symptoms and signs of decreased blood volume (flat neck veins, postural changes in blood pressure, elevated hematocrit, lowered hourly urine volume).

(Frame 42)

Fluid orders should be rewritten every _____ hours and should include _____ allowances and correction allowances in this order: water, _____ , acid-base, and _____ .

Saline excess usually occurs in patients with cirrhosis, protein depletion, or cardiac insufficiency; its main signs are edema and weight gain. In both saline depletion and excess, the serum Na^+ concentration is _____ (raised/lowered/normal).

(Frame 43)

You should first consider the patient's maintenance allowances, the amount of fluid and electrolytes needed to replace anticipated daily losses. Then formulate any correction allowances in this order: water, saline, acid-base, and potassium.

(Frame 95)

normal

Treatment for saline depletion is administration of isotonic saline; treatment for saline excess consists of restriction of salt and administration of diuretics.

(Frame 44)

This section will list a program to follow each day of a patient's stay in the hospital. Each patient's fluid requirements should be reevaluated every _____ hours.

(Frame 94)

The most common combined saline and water imbalance is saline depletion and water excess, where, for instance, an athlete perspires profusely and then drinks an excessive amount of water. Treatment involves administration of saline or, in the above case, salt tablets.

PART V

Applications

(Frame 93)

A sensitive yet easy method for assessing changes in saline status over a period of time (during a hospital stay) is based on change in body weight (Δ body weight). Any change in saline is reflected in the _____ fluid space.

capacity
excess

4. Serum K^+ reflects potassium metabolism: high in K^+ excess, low in K^+ depletion.
5. Note rules on giving potassium.

extracellular

Two additional factors in this calculation are water of metabolism and change in water status. The first adds fluid to the extracellular space and is figured by multiplying 0.3 kg/day kg/day times the number of days considered.

SUMMARY

1. Total body potassium equal to potassium capacity: normal
2. Total body potassium less than potassium _____ : potassium depletion
3. Total body potassium greater than potassium capacity: potassium
   _____

The second factor, change in water status, must be accounted for, due to its effect on intracellular volume. It is calculated by multiplying the percentage change in Na^+ times intracellular volume (40 percent $\times$ body weight for the average person).

(Frame 48)

cardiac

IV HCO_3^- raises the blood pH and lowers serum K^+. IV glucose and insulin lower serum K^+ by adding to potassium capacity (deposition of glycogen). Emergency peritoneal dialysis should follow, if needed.

(Frame 90)

The complete formula is:

$$\Delta \text{ extracellular volume} = \Delta \text{ body weight}$$

$$+$$

$$(0.3) \times (\text{days})$$

$$\pm$$

$$(\%\Delta \text{ Na}^+) \times (40\%) \times (\text{body weight}).$$

(Frame 49)

irreversible cardiac arrhythmias

Potassium excess causes EKG changes which may progress to _____ arrest. IV calcium should first be given, just fast enough to maintain a normal EKG. The next steps actually lower serum K^+.

For example, if a 75 kg man checks into the hospital with his Na^+ equal to 140, but 5 days later is found to be 73 kg with a Na^+ of 130, his change in extracellular volume (ECV) is:

$\Delta ECV = -2 \ (\Delta \ \text{body weight})$

$+0.3 \times 5 \ (\text{water of} \ \underline{\hspace{6cm}} \ )$

$- (140 - 130)/130 \times 0.4 \times 75 \ (\text{change in water status})$

$= -2.8$ liters (saline depletion).

24
40
50
240

4. Never give more than _____ mEq K^+ in any one-hour period.

A mistake here could cause _____ _____

_____ .

(Frame 88)

1. Water depletion—signs: mental dysfunction, thirst, concentrated urine; treatment: give water
2. Water excess—signs: mental dysfunction, oliguria; treatment: restrict water
3. Saline depletion—history: loss of sodium containing fluid; signs: flat neck veins, postural changes in blood pressure, elevated hematocrit, lowered hourly urine volume; treatment: give saline

Review of rules for administering K^+:

1. Reevaluate need every _____ hours.
2. IV fluids should never contain more than _____ mEq/liter K^+.
3. Never attempt more than a _____ percent correction of potassium depletion in one 24 hour period; even then, do not exceed _____ mEq in this time interval.

(Frame 87)

4. Saline excess—history: cirrhosis, protein depletion, or cardiac insufficiency; signs: edema, weight gain; treatment: salt restriction, diuretics
5. Assess subtle changes in saline status over time:

$$\Delta \text{ EVC} = (\Delta \text{ body weight}) + (0.3 \times \text{days}) \pm (\%\Delta \text{Na}^+ \times 0.4 \times \text{body weight}).$$

4. Never give more than 20 mEq K^+ in any one-hour period.

A mistake here could cause irreversible cardiac arrhythmias.

(Frame 86)

PART III

Acid-Base Disturbances

(Frame 53)

Rules for administering potassium:

1. Reevaluate need every 24 hours.
2. IV fluids should never contain more than 40 mEq/liter K^+.
3. Never attempt more than a 50 percent correction of potassium depletion in one 24-hour period; even then, do not exceed 240 mEq in this time interval.

(Frame 85)

The pH (negative logarithm of H^+ concentration) best expresses the body's acid-base status and is intimately related to the disposition of carbonic acid:

$$CO_2 + H_2O \;\rightleftharpoons\; H_2CO_3 \;\rightleftharpoons\; H^+ + HCO_3$$

carbonic acid

(Frame 54)

Finally, percentage depletion is multiplied by potassium capacity to get K^+ deficit in milliequivalents. A 70 kg normal male therefore has $45 \times 70 = 3{,}150$ mEq potassium capacity (see Frame 81). A 10 percent deficit means he needs $0.10 \times 3{,}150 = 315$ mEq K^+.

(Frame 84)

The pH is most easily interpreted by means of the Henderson-Hasselbalch equation:

$$pH = 6.1 + \log \frac{HCO_3^-}{P_{CO_2}}$$

pH is dependent upon the ratio of bicarbonate to CO_2 tension: "As goes the ratio, so goes the pH."

(Frame 55)

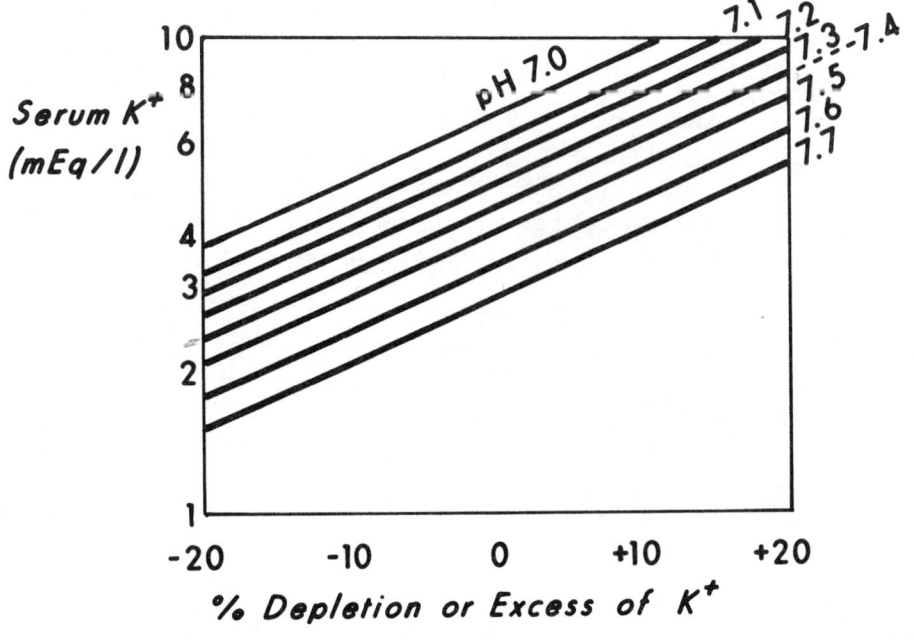

(Frame 83)

That is, if the ratio rises, the pH rises; if the ratio falls, the pH _____.
The normal pH range is 7.35 to 7.45, although a diseased patient can live from pH 6.9 to pH 7.6. HCO_3^- is normally 25 to 30 mEq/liter and P_{CO_2}, 35 to 45 mm Hg.

Second, the percentage of depletion is estimated using the nomogram in the following frame (pH and serum K^+ must be known).

falls

In referring back to the reactions in Frame 54, you can see that CO_2 and HCO_3^- sit on opposite sides of carbonic acid, and that an excess or deficit of either will change the H^+ concentration (and, of course, the pH). It is the ratio of the two that determines the

——————————————— .

(Frame 57)

total

Potassium capacity in mEq/kg body weight, estimated from degree of wasting:

	Males	Females
Normal	45 mEq/kg	35 mEq/kg
Moderate wasting	32 mEq/kg	25 mEq/kg
Marked wasting	23 mEq/kg	20 mEq/kg

(Frame 81)

pH

If you know any two of the three values of pH, P_{CO_2}, of HCO_3^-, you can find the other by using the nomogram in the next frame. "As goes the ratio, so goes the pH."

Potassium depletion is treated by giving K^+ so as to match the _____ body potassium to the potassium capacity. The amount to give is calculated by first determining the potassium capacity using the table in the next frame.

(Frame 80)

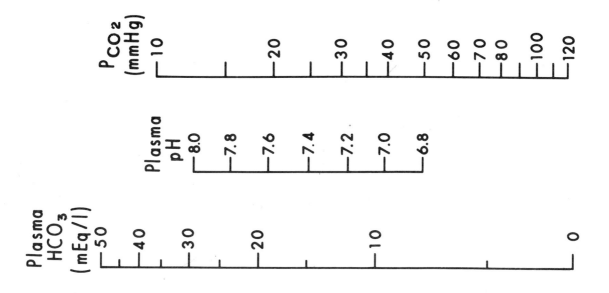

P_{CO_2}
(mmHg)

10 — 20 — 30 — 40 — 50 — 60 — 70 — 80 — 100 — 120

Plasma
pH

8.0 — 7.8 — 7.6 — 7.4 — 7.2 — 7.0 — 6.8

Plasma
HCO_3
(mEq/l)

50 — 40 — 30 — 20 — 10 — 0

(Frame 59)

falling

In diseases involving long-term wasting, much tissue can be broken down; however, as long as total body potassium equals potassium capacity, serum K^+ will be normal, indicating normal potassium metabolism. This is true although a great deal of potassium can be lost from the body.

(Frame 79)

The two main mechanisms by which the body protects pH are action of body buffers and excretion of H^+.

The serum K^+ reflects changes in potassium metabolism, rising with potassium excess and _____ with potassium depletion. Serum K^+ is normally 3.8 to 4.4 mEq/liter.

The body buffers, all of which are in equilibrium with each other, include the H_2CO_3/HCO_3^- system, hemoglobin, tissue proteins, and bone. The status of one buffer reflects the status of the others, since they are in _____ with each other.

Potassium depletion is defined as a total body potassium less than the potassium capacity; this condition occurs from a loss of K^+ in diarrhea or during diuretic therapy.

Potassium excess is defined as a total body potassium _____ (less/more) than the potassium capacity; it occurs in renal failure.

(Frame 77)

equilibrium

H$^+$ excretion is carried out mainly by the kidney through the attachment of H$^+$ to sulfate and phosphate ions and to ammonia. The body buffers act first in adjusting the pH. Excretion of _____ backs up these buffers and even forms more HCO$_3^-$: H$_2$CO$_3$ $\rightarrow$ HCO$_3^-$ + H$^+$ (excreted).

Potassium (K^+) is essentially an intracellular ion, and as such it is associated with negatively charged anions (PO_4^{3-}, proteins) collectively called the potassium capacity. During normal metabolism, total body potassium equals potassium capacity.

H^+

Acid-base disorders arise through metabolic means (change in HCO_3^-) or through respiratory means (change in P_{CO_2}). "As goes the _____ so goes the _____ ."

PART IV

Potassium Imbalances

(Frame 75)

ratio
pH

One can derive the four primary acid-base disorders by examining the HCO_3^-/P_{CO_2} ratio (see Henderson-Hasselbalch equation in Frame 55):

1. $\downarrow HCO_3^-/P_{CO_2}$ —$\downarrow$pH—metabolic acidosis
2. $\uparrow HCO_3^-/P_{CO_2}$ —$\uparrow$pH—metabolic alkalosis
3. $HCO_3^-/\uparrow P_{CO_2}$ —$\downarrow$pH—respiratory acidosis
4. $HCO_3^-/\downarrow P_{CO_2}$ —$\uparrow$pH—respiratory alkalosis

(Frame 64)

ratio
pH

5. Four primary disorders are:

   a. Metabolic acidosis—$\downarrow HCO_3^-$
   b. Metabolic alkalosis—$\uparrow HCO_3^-$
   c. Respiratory acidosis—$\uparrow P_{CO_2}$
   d. Respiratory alkalosis—$\downarrow P_{CO_2}$

(Frame 74)

Fill in the following table:

1. $\uparrow HCO_3^- /P_{CO_2}$ —metabolic _____
2. $HCO_3^- /\uparrow P_{CO_2}$ —respiratory_____
3. $\downarrow HCO_3^- /P_{CO_2}$ —_____
4. $HCO_3^- /\downarrow P_{CO_2}$ —_____

(Frame 65)

SUMMARY

1. Acid-base status is reflected by pH

2. $CO_2 + H_2O \rightleftharpoons H_2CO_3 \rightleftharpoons H^+ + HCO_3^-$

3. $pH = 6.1 + \log HCO_3^-/P_{CO_2}$

4. "As goes the _____ , so goes the _____."

5. Acid-base status is defended by body buffers and excretion of H^+.

1. alkalosis
2. acidosis
3. metabolic acidosis
4. respiratory alkalosis

Metabolic acidosis arises due to removal of HCO_3^- by loss of alkaline fluids (diarrhea, intestinal suction) or by addition of H^+ (aspirin poisoning, diabetic acidosis, renal failure). In all these cases, the ratio in the Henderson-Hasselbalch equation is _____ (increased/decreased).

(Frame 66)

decrease
increase

Extraneous (and confusing) nomenclature includes the following:

1. Plasma CO_2 tension = P_{CO_2}
2. CO_2 combining power = HCO_3^-
3. Plasma CO_2 content = $HCO_3^- + P_{CO_2}$

(Frame 72)

decreased

Metabolic acidosis is treated by administration of HCO_3^-, in the amount determined by the following formula:

HCO_3^-, mEq = (3) × (ECV in liters) × (desired change in HCO_3^-).

If you want to raise the HCO_3^- of a 75 kg man (ECV = 15 liters) by 5 mEq/liter, give him 3 × 15 × 5 = 225 mEq HCO_3^-.

(Frame 67)

Respiratory alkalosis is caused by hyperventilation (anxiety, fever), reflected by a
_____ in P_{CO_2} and an _____ in the
ratio. One should treat the underlying disease in this disorder.

(Frame 71)

Metabolic alkalosis occurs when the renal threshold for HCO_3^- is raised, thus raising the HCO_3^- to high levels (the ratio is therefore _____).

Chloride depletion and potassium depletion are the main causes of metabolic alkalosis, and these are treated with potassium and sodium chloride.

(Frame 68)

increased

Respiratory acidosis is due to ventilatory impairment of a variety of causes (pulmonary disease, rib fixation) and is treated by improving ventilation, not by fluid therapy. The ratio goes down because the P_{CO_2} goes _____ .

To continue, turn the text over.

(Frame 69)